LOW-HISTAMINE DIETING COOKBOOK

Tasty and Delicious Recipes for Beginners

Fighting with Histamine Intolerance

TABLE OF CONTENT

PREFACE

In the journey to optimal health, understanding your body's responses and catering to its unique needs becomes paramount.

Histamine intolerance, often underestimated, can significantly impact one's well-being. This cookbook aims to guide you through the intricacies of histamine intolerance, illuminate the importance of adopting a low-histamine diet, and provide a treasure trove of delectable recipes tailored to nourish and delight.

Know that navigating a low-histamine lifestyle doesn't mean sacrificing flavor and satisfaction. This cookbook is your companion on the path to wellness, offering a diverse array of mouthwatering recipes meticulously crafted to be low in histamine yet high in taste.

From breakfast delights to sumptuous dinners, snacks, and indulgent desserts, each recipe is a celebration of wholesome ingredients and culinary creativity.

I understand the challenges of adopting a new dietary approach, and my goal is to make your journey enjoyable and sustainable. Beyond recipes, you'll find practical tips, kitchen essentials, and special occasion menus to guide you through every aspect of embracing a low-histamine lifestyle.

Embark on this culinary adventure with us, and discover that a low-histamine diet can be a journey of delicious possibilities. Your health and happiness are at the heart of this cookbook, and we invite you to savor every moment of this transformative experience.

INTRODUCTION

The body depends on histamine, a naturally occurring chemical found in various foods, for numerous essential functions. On the other hand, some individuals may develop histamine intolerance as a result of an imbalance. A more refined approach to one's diet is necessary due to the potential emergence of symptoms such as skin irritations, migraines, and gastrointestinal problems.

I will provide you with comprehensive knowledge about histamine intoxication as we explore this subject, enabling you to make informed decisions regarding your dietary choices.

Choosing to embrace a low-carbohydrate diet goes beyond mere adjustments to one's eating routine; it represents a transformative step towards improved well-being. Reducing the consumption of sodium-rich foods can have a positive impact on symptoms and overall well-being. This dietary change is not just a passing trend; it's a unique approach to enhancing well-being and balance in one's life.

This book seeks to analyze histamine intolerance and the scientific principles behind it, highlighting the significant impact of diet in managing its symptoms.

Histamine, an organic molecule, can be found in both the human body and various types of food. It plays a role in over a dozen different physiological activities. It controls a wide range of tasks as a neurotransmitter, including digestion, immune response, and sleep-wake cycles. However, some individuals experience a blending that can result in a lack of tolerance.

This ailment arises from an imbalance in histamine production within the body, leading to a range of symptoms such as rashes, headaches, gastrointestinal issues, and other related manifestations. A thorough comprehension of the origins of histamine is crucial in effectively addressing intolerance.

CHAPTER ONE

One critical component of a low-histamine diet is reducing foods that are high in histamine or cause histamine to be released. To manage your symptoms by carefully selecting ingredients and cooking procedures. Generally, this approach consists of:

Choosing Fresh Foods

Choosing fresh, unprocessed food helps reduce histamine consumption. A low-histamine diet emphasizes fresh fruits, vegetables, and lean proteins. Avoiding High-Heat Foods: Identifying and reducing high-heat foods such as aged cheeses, cured meats, and fermented products is vital.

Understanding Histamine Liberators

Some foods do not contain histamine but can promote its release in the body. Some examples include specific foods, alcohol, and some fruits.

Mindful Cooking Techniques

Cooking methods such as grilling, frying, and frying can raise histamine levels in foods. Using gentler cooking methods, such as steaming or boiling, can be beneficial.

Reading Labels

Learning to read food labels is necessary. Artificial preservatives and additives might raise histamine levels.

FOODS HIGH IN HISTAMINE

To successfully start a low-histamine diet, one must be well-versed in the several foods that are rich in this neurotransmitter.

I will provide you with a comprehensive rundown of all the foods that are commonly linked to elevated histam ine levels.

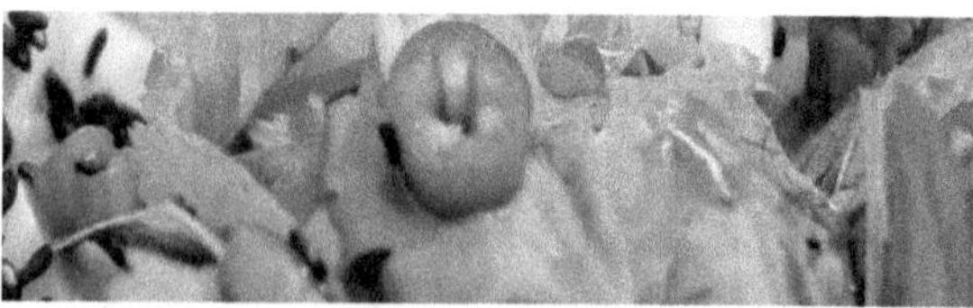

Because everyone has a different tolerance level, some people can have a strong reaction to foods that are high in histamine, while others can tolerate them in moderate amounts.

People have various tolerances, therefore it's important to remember that.

Aged Cheeses

Cheese lovers, you should take heed. Numerous aged cheeses, including cheddar, gouda, and parmesan, are filled with a significant amount of histamine. Consider the possibility of experimenting with fresh cheeses such as mozzarella or goat cheese as alternatives.

Processed and Cured Meats

In spite of their delectable taste, processed and cured meats are widely recognized for the high levels of heinousness that they contain. Among the most common offender types are bacon, salami, ham, and sausages. Reduce your consumption of histamine by selecting fresh cuts of meat that are low in fat.

Fermented Foods

Fermentation, despite being praised for its positive effects on health, might be problematic for individuals who have a problem with stomach insufficiency. For instance, sauerkraut, kischles, pickles, and soy sauce are all examples. Participate in the experience of preparing handmade variations with shorter preparation periods.

Vinegar and Vinegar-Containing Foods

Vinegar, which is commonly found in kitchens, is categorized as a histamine liberator. Not only does this encompass the condiment itself, but it also encompasses other meals and dressings that use vinegar. You might want to think about using lemon or lime juice as alternatives.

Alcoholic Beverages

Certain alcoholic beverages, including red wine, beer, and champagne, have the potential to induce histamine release within the body.

Among the available possibilities, clear spirits such as vodka and gin might be more well-tolerated.

Certain Fruits

There are some fruits that are high in histamine, despite the fact that fruits are generally healthy. A few examples of such fruits include strawberries, bananas, pineapples, and citrus fruits. Consider selecting alternatives that have a lower heart rate, such as apples, pears, or berries.

Tomatoes and Tomato-Based Products

Due to the presence of histamine, tomatoes, which are a common ingredient in a wide variety of meals, can be problematic. This encompasses products that 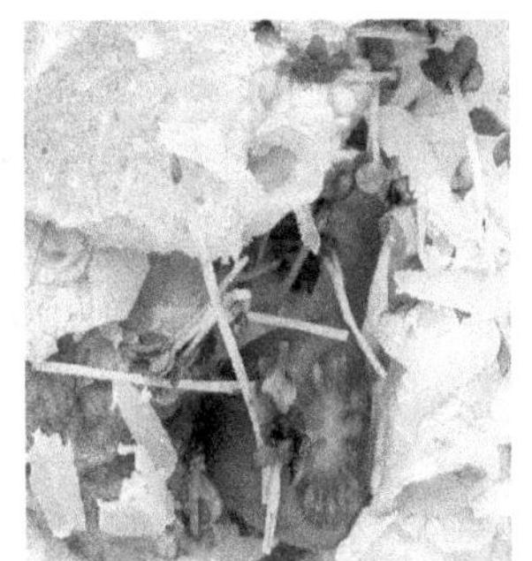 are derived from tomatoes, such as ketchup and sauces. Make an effort to utilize fresh alternatives such as red bell peppers.

Shellfish

Those who enjoy seafood should exercise caution because shellfish, including shrimp, crab, and lobster, contain a significant amount of hexamine. You might want to think about selecting fresh fish varieties such as salmon or cod.

Spinach and Eggplant

There are particular vegetables, such as spinach and eggplant, that have higher levels of histamine. Experiment with other alternative options that are rich in nutrients, such as kale, zucchini, or broccoli.

Chocolate and Cocoa Products

In individuals who possess a sweet tooth, the presence of chlorate can be a challenge because of its high histamine content. Treats or desserts that are based on carbohydrates and contain low levels of histamine should be explored.

When one begins to adopt a lifestyle that is low in histamine, it is not merely a matter of making adjustments to one's dietary choices; rather, it is a transformative journey that presents numerous opportunities for overall well-being.

Mitigating Histamine Intolerance Symptoms

The condition known as hypertension is frequently linked to recurrent headaches and migraines. Individuals frequently report a reduction in the frequency and intensity of these debilitating symptoms when they significantly reduce the amount of foods that are high in histamine.

Improved Digestive Health

Issues related to digestion, including but not limited to bleeding, abdominal pain, and irregular bowel movements, have been associated with histamine instability.

A diet that is low in carbohydrates can contribute to a digestive system that is more tranquil, which in turn promotes regularity and comfort.

Enhanced Skin Health

The presence of histamine is known to be a factor in skin-related issues such as hives, itching, and eczema. It is possible that adopting a lifestyle that is low in histamine could result in a significant improvement in skin health, thereby alleviating these discomforts and promoting a more streamlined understanding.

Balanced Energy Levels

The changes in histamine levels have the potential to cause energy surges and crashes. As a result of the regulation of histamine intake, individuals frequently report experiencing increased levels of consistent energy, hence reducing feelings of fatigue and lethargy.

Improved Sleep Quality

The hormone histamine is involved in the process of regulating the sleep-wake cycle. It is possible for those who have histamine intolerance to experience disturbances when they are sleeping. Having a lifestyle that is low in stress may contribute to a more peaceful and refreshing sleep, which in turn can help to improve overall wellness.

Supporting Mental Well-Being

It is possible for histamine intolerance to have an impact on cognitive function, which can result in symptoms that are usually referred to as "brain fog." When individuals follow a diet that is low in sodium, they frequently report experiencing an increase in mental clarity and focus.

Mood swings and irritability are something that may be experienced by certain persons who have a sensitivity to gluten. An individual who adopts a lifestyle that is low in histamine may experience a more stable and positive emotional state.

Allergy Management

Hormone insufficiency has the potential to mimic the symptoms of allergic reactions, which may include nasal congestion, itching, and watery eyes. It is possible for individuals to experience a reduction in these allergy-like signs by reducing the consumption of foods that are high in histamine.

Overall Inflammation Reduction

Chronic inflammation has been associated with a wide range of health concerns. In order to promote long-term health, adopting a lifestyle that is low in histamines can potentially lead to a reduction in overall inflammatory indicators. This is achieved by avoiding the consumption of foods that contribute to inflammation.

Individualized Approach to Nutrition

Individuals are encouraged to become more in tune with their bodies and to make dietary decisions that are tailored to their specific needs when they choose a low-heat lifestyle. Having this awareness allows for a more profound connection to be established with one's dietary requirements and preferences.

Long-Term Health and Wellness

When a low-height lifestyle is maintained over a period of time, it can be considered a proactive approach for ensuring long-term health to be maintained. Individuals can effectively contribute to their overall well-being and potentially minimize the risk of certain health issues by managing their histamine intake.

CHAPTER TWO

LOW-HISTAMINE RECIPES

All of the recipes in this carefully compiled cookbook are suitable for anyone following a low-carbohydrate diet, and they include a wide variety of foods, from main courses to sweets.

These recipes have been carefully crafted, and I hope you'll take the time to explore and enjoy them. The delectable delights of sweets, the satisfying meals, and the imaginative treats for kids all fall under this category. Inspiring recipes that put your health first without compromising on taste will be revealed as you delve further into each section.

You can see how versatile low-histamine components are and how much room for imagination there is in each recipe by looking at them individually.

No matter your level of experience in the kitchen, we aim to offer a variety of recipes that are both nutritious and enjoyable to make and share with those you care about.

Energizing Smoothie Bowl

Ingredients

Smoothie Base

- 1 cup fresh mixed berries (blueberries, strawberries, raspberries)
- 1 ripe banana, peeled and sliced
- 1/2 cup diced pineapple (fresh or frozen)
- 1/2 cup unsweetened almond milk or coconut milk
- 1 tablespoon chia seeds (optional for added texture and nutrition)
- 1 teaspoon honey or maple syrup (optional for sweetness)

Toppings

- Sliced fresh fruits (kiwi, strawberries, banana)
- Granola or gluten-free oats
- Coconut flakes
- Chopped nuts (almonds, walnuts)
- Fresh mint leaves for garnish

Instructions

- Put the mixed berries, the sliced banana, the diced pineapple, the almond milk, the chia seeds (if you are using them), and the honey or maple syrup into a blender and blend until smooth.
- Blend until smooth and creamy, adjusting the consistency by adding additional almond milk if necessary. Blend until smooth and creamy.
- The smoothie should be poured into a bowl, ensuring that it has a smooth and even surface finish.

- An arrangement of sliced fresh fruits, granola or oats, coconut flakes, and chopped nuts should be arranged on top of the basis of the smoothie.

- Take advantage of your creative abilities to create a visually appealing arrangement for your bowl.

- The bowl should be garnished with fresh mint leaves to add a splash of color and an additional layer of freshness.

- Grab a spoon and take the time to appreciate the vibrant flavors and textures that your energizing smoothie bowl has to offer.

- The process of mixing and matching the bites allows one to experience a combination of the sweetness of fruit, the crunchiness of granola, and the creaminess of the smoothie base.

Low-Histamine Oatmeal

Ingredients

- 1 cup rolled oats (gluten-free oats for those with gluten sensitivity)
- 2 cups water or low-histamine milk alternative (almond milk, coconut milk)
- 1-2 tablespoons honey or maple syrup (optional, adjust to taste)
- 1 teaspoon vanilla extract for added flavor (ensure it's low in alcohol content)

Instructions

- Put the rolled oats and liquid (either water or milk alternative) into a saucepan and mix them together properly.
- As the mixture is heated over medium heat, whisk it occasionally while it is being brought to a gentle boil.
- As soon as the water boils, reduce the heat to a low level and allow the oats to cool down.

Strive to stir occasionally in order to avoid sticking.

- You can add honey or maple syrup to the oats if you want to make them sweeter. You can adjust the sweetness to suit your preferences in terms of taste.

- In order to enhance the flavor, stir the mixture in a vanilla extract. It is imperative to ensure that the vanilla extract has a low alcohol concentration in order to comply with the standards for low-heat.

- You should continue to consume the oats for around five to ten minutes, or until the oats reach the desired consistency. For some individuals, a creamier texture is more appealing, while others prefer a little stiffer bite.

Scrumptious Breakfast Muffins

Ingredients

Dry Ingredients

- 1 ½ cups oat flour (gluten-free if needed)
- ½ cup almond flour
- 1 teaspoon baking powder
- ½ teaspoon baking soda
- ¼ teaspoon salt

Wet Ingredients

- 2 ripe bananas, mashed
- 2 large eggs
- ½ cup low-histamine milk alternative (almond milk, coconut milk)
- ¼ cup maple syrup or honey
- ¼ cup melted coconut oil or other low-histamine oil
- 1 teaspoon vanilla extract (ensure low alcohol content)

Add-ins

- ½ cup fresh blueberries or diced strawberries
- ¼ cup chopped nuts (walnuts or almonds)
- ¼ cup shredded coconut

Instructions

- The oven should be preheated to 350 degrees Fahrenheit (175 degrees Celsius). You may either use paper liners to line a muffin tin or you can glaze the muffin cups.
- Put the oat flour, almond flour, baking powder, baking soda, and salt into a large mixing bowl and mix them together. While working together till they are well integrated.
- An additional bowl should be used to mash the ripe bananas. Make sure to incorporate the eggs, a low-fat milk option, maple syrup or honey, melted coconut oil, and vanilla extract into the mixture. Ensure that the wet elements are well combined by thoroughly mixing them together.

- It is necessary to pour the liquid ingredients into the bowl that contains the dry ingredients. Gently combine the ingredients by folding them together until they are completely combined. It is important to avoid overmixing in order to maintain a texture that is more stable.

- Caution should be exercised when incorporating fresh blueberries or diced strawberries, chopped nuts, and shredded coconut into the mixture. Distribute them in this manner. all the way through the batter.

- Take the batter and pour it into the prepared muffle cups, making sure that each one is approximately two-thirds filled.

- You should position the muffin tin in the preheated oven and bake it for around 18 to 20 minutes, or until a toothpick that is inserted into the center comes out clean.

- Make sure to allow the muffins to cool down in the container for a few minutes before transferring them to a wire rack to finish cooling down entirely.

- You have the liberty to personalize the muffins by adding additional toppings such as a sprinkling of oats, a drizzle of honey, or a dusting of powdered sugar.

- For a few days, store the Scrumptious Breakfast Muffins in an airtight container at room temperature. Alternatively, refrigerate them for a longer period of time to ensure continuous freshness.

Ingredients

- 4 cups mixed salad greens (baby spinach, arugula, kale, or a combination)
- 1 cup cherry tomatoes, halved
- 1 cucumber, thinly sliced
- 1 bell pepper (red, yellow, or orange), diced
- 1 cup radishes, thinly sliced
- 1 cup grilled chicken breast, sliced
- 1/2 cup chickpeas (canned and rinsed)
- 1/2 cup crumbled feta or goat cheese (low-histamine options)
- 1/4 cup toasted pine nuts or slivered almonds
- 1/4 cup extra-virgin olive oil
- 2 tablespoons balsamic vinegar (ensure low-histamine)
- 1 teaspoon Dijon mustard
- 1 teaspoon honey (optional, for sweetness)
- Salt and pepper to taste

Instructions

- Ensure that the salad greens are thoroughly washed and dried. Place the ingredients in a large salad bowl.

- Ensure that the cherry tomatoes, sliced cucumber, diced bell pepper, and sliced red onions are all included in the mixture. Combine thoroughly in order to distribute the vegetables in an even manner.

- Make sure to arrange the sliced chicken breast and chicken breasts that have been grilled on top of the greens. By incorporating a protein boost, this enhances the filling capacity of the salad.

- Consider topping the salad with crumbled cheese or goat cheese if you are in the mood for a cheese-based dish. Select options that are low in histamine to accommodate your dietary requirements.

- For a delectable crunch, you can toast pine nuts or almonds according to your preference.

In order to enhance the flavor and texture of the salad, sprinkle them over it.

- In a small bowl, combine the extra-virgin olive oil, balsamic vinegar, Dijon mustard, honey (if using), salt, and pepper. Whisk all of these ingredients together until uniform. The sweetness and seasoning should be adjusted to suit your personal preferences in terms of taste.

- Ensure that the home-made dressing is drizzled over the salad, ensuring that it is evenly covered. To ensure that every ingredient is evenly coated with the flavorful dressing, gently toss the salad.

- PtsPlease serve the flavorful and fresh food. Salad immediately, enabling everyone to take pleasure in the vibrant colors and textures that are present.

Sandwiches and Wraps

Ingredients

- Whole-grain bread slices or gluten-free wraps
- Sliced turkey or chicken breast (low-histamine)
- Smoked salmon or canned tuna (low-histamine)
- Fresh lettuce leaves
- Sliced tomatoes
- Cucumber, thinly sliced
- Avocado, sliced
- Spreads and Condiments:
- Hummus or tahini
- Dijon mustard or a low-histamine mayo
- Pesto made with low-histamine ingredients
- Cheese (Optional):
- Sliced low-histamine cheese (cheddar, Swiss, or goat cheese)
- Sprouts or microgreens for added freshness and crunch

Instructions

- While making your sandwich or wrap, choose whole-grain bread slices or glute-free wraps as the base for your sandwich or wrap.

- A layer of hummus, tahini, Dijon mustard, or low-sodium mayonnaise can be spread on the bread or wrap in order to add a flavorful base.

- Place fresh lettuce leaves on the base for a crisp and refreshing layer.

- To enhance the flavor of the greens, arrange slices of turkey, chicken, smoked salmon, or canned tuna on top of the greens. Please make sure that the sources of protein are low in sodium.

- If you want to add a splash of color, taste, and nutrients to your dish, layer sliced tomatoes, cucumbers, and avocados first.

- If desired, you can incorporate a layer of sliced low-fat cheese to enhance the creaminess and richness of the dish.

- In order to achieve an additional layer of flavor, drizzle a pesto that is created with low-histamine ingredients over another layer of ingredients.

- For an additional layer of freshness and a wonderful crunch, sprinkle some sprouts or microgreens on top of the dish.

- In order to create wraps, it is necessary to fold the sides and roll them tightly. When preparing sandwiches, lay the second slice of bread on top and gently push it down.

- PtsTo create an elegant presentation, you can either slice the sandwich or wrap it diagonally. Be prepared with toothpicks in the event that they are required.

Lemon Baked Chicken

Ingredients

- 4 boneless, skinless chicken breasts
- 1/4 cup olive oil
- 1/4 cup fresh lemon juice (approximately 2 lemons)
- 2 cloves garlic, minced
- 1 teaspoon dried oregano

- 1 teaspoon dried thyme
- 1 teaspoon dried rosemary
- Salt and pepper to taste
- Lemon slices for garnish
- Fresh parsley, chopped, for garnish

Instructions

- The oven should be preheated to 400 degrees Fahrenheit (200 degrees Celsius).
- It is recommended to use paper towels to dry the chicken breasts. Put them in a plastic bag that can be sealed back up or a shallow dish for the purpose of marinating.
- Olive oil, fresh lemon juice, minced garlic, dried oregano, dried thyme, dried rosemary, salt, and pepper should be mixed together in a bowl using a whisk. Check that the marinade is thoroughly mixed together.
- Spread the marinade evenly over the chicken breasts, making sure that each individual piece is thoroughly coated. Marinate the ingredients in the refrigerator for a minimum of thirty

minutes, allowing the flavors to develop more fully.

- Ensure that the chicken breasts that have been marinated are transferred to a baking dish and arranged in a single layer.

- For approximately 25 to 30 minutes, or until the internal temperature of the chicken reaches 165 degrees Fahrenheit (74 degrees Celsius), bake the chicken in the preheated oven. It is possible for the baking times to differ depending on the thickness of the chicken breasts.

- For optimal flavor and texture, it is recommended to basting the chicken with the juices from the pan as it is being baked.

- To achieve a skin that is golden and crispy, you have the option of broiling the chicken for an extra two to three minutes at the conclusion of the cooking period. It is important to maintain a close eye in order to avoid experiencing burns.

- To guarantee that the chicken is fully cooked, it is advisable to utilize a meat thermometer.

When the juices are poured, they should be clear, and there should be no pink color in the middle.

- A vivid finish can be achieved by garnishing the Lemon Baked Chicken with fresh lemon slices and chopped parsley when it is served. Enjoy it while it's still hot!

Shrimp and Broccoli Stir-Fry

Ingredients

- 1 pound large shrimp, peeled and deveined
- 3 cups broccoli florets
- 1 red bell pepper, sliced
- 1 carrot, julienned
- 3 green onions, chopped (separate white and green parts)
- 1/4 cup soy sauce (low-sodium)
- 2 tablespoons oyster sauce
- 1 tablespoon hoisin sauce
- 1 tablespoon sesame oil
- 1 tablespoon rice vinegar
- 1 tablespoon honey or brown sugar

- 3 cloves garlic, minced

- 1 tablespoon ginger, grated

- 2 tablespoons vegetable oil (for cooking)

Garnish (Optional):

- Sesame seeds

- Chopped cilantro

Instructions

- The shrimp should be patted dry with paper towels and then set aside.

- A bowl should be used to combine soy sauce, oyster sauce, hoisin sauce, sesame oil, rice vinegar, and honey (or brown sugar). The mixture should be whisked together. Obtain a seat.

- Prepare the vegetable oil by heating it in a large wok or skillet over a medium-high heat.

- When the oil is hot, add grated ginger and minced garlic to it. Stir the mixture for around thirty seconds till it becomes fragrant.

- Add the shrimp to the pan and allow them to cook for around two to three minutes, or until they begin to turn pink. Taking the shrimp out of the pan, remove them and set them aside.

- In the same pan, if additional oil is required, add it into the pan. Incorporate the brussels sprouts, red bell pepper, carrot, and the white parts of the green onions when stirring. Stir-fry the vegetables for three to four minutes, during which time they should be somewhat tender but still crisp.

- Ensure that the cooked shrimp is returned to the pan together with the vegetables.

- It is recommended to pour the prepared sauce over the shrimp and vegetables. Stir everything thoroughly to ensure that it is completely coated.

- You should continue cooking for a further two to three minutes until the shrimp are completely cooked and the sauce has become somewhat thickened.

- In the event that preferred, garnish the Shrimp and Broccoli Stir-Fry with the green parts of the chopped onions, the same seeds, and chopped cilantro.

- Ensure that the stir-fry is served over a seasoned rice, noodles, or your preferred foundation while it is still serving hot. Have fun!!

One-Pot Lentil and Vegetable Stew

Ingredients

- 1 cup dried brown or green lentils, rinsed and drained

- 1 onion, diced

- 2 carrots, peeled and diced

- 2 celery stalks, chopped

- 3 garlic cloves, minced

- 1 bell pepper (red, yellow, or green), diced

- 1 zucchini, diced

- 1 sweet potato, peeled and diced

- 1 can (14 oz) diced tomatoes

- 1 can (6 oz) tomato paste
- 6 cups vegetable or low-sodium vegetable broth
- 2 bay leaves
- 1 teaspoon ground cumin
- 1 teaspoon ground coriander
- 1 teaspoon smoked paprika
- 1/2 teaspoon turmeric
- Salt and pepper to taste
- 2 cups chopped kale or spinach
- 2 tablespoons olive oil
- Fresh parsley, chopped

Instructions

- The process involves heating olive oil in a big pot or Dutch oven over medium heat. Include diced onion, carrots, celery, and garlic in the mixture. Sauté the vegetables for five to seven minutes till they get tender.
- Combine ground cumin, ground coriander, smoked paprika, turmeric, salt, and pepper in a bowl and stir until combined. To toast the

spices, continue cooking for an additional one to two minutes.

- Make sure to add the rinsed lentils to the pot and stir them so that they are coated with the organic mixture.

- While stirring, incorporate the diced tomatoes and tomato paste into the mixture. This will ensure that the lentils and vegetables are thoroughly combined.

- Include the bell pepper, zucchini, and sweet potato in the dish that has been diced. Stir thoroughly in order to ensure that the ingredients are distributed equally.

- The mixture should be brought to a gentle boil after the addition of bay leaves and the addition of vegetable broth.

- Reduce the temperature to a low level, cover the pot, and allow the soil to warm up for a period of twenty-five to thirty minutes, or until the leaves and vegetables have become tender. On occasion, stir the mixture.

- Once you have tasted the stew, adjust the seasoning if necessary by adding additional salt or pepper according to your personal preference.

- You can add chopped spinach or chopped kale to the saucepan in the final five minutes of cooking if you are using it. Stir the mixture until the greens have evaporated.

- The bay leaves should be discarded prior to serving.

- To prepare the One-Pot Label and Vegetable Stew, place the ingredients into bowls. Depending on your preference, garnish with chopped fresh parsley.

- Please ensure that the stew is served hot, possibly accompanied by a side of crusty bread or a dollop of Greek yogurt.

Cucumber Hummus Bites

Ingredients

- 2 large English cucumbers
- 1 cup homemade or store-bought hummus
- Cherry tomatoes, halved
- Kalamata olives, pitted and sliced
- Feta cheese, crumbled
- Fresh parsley, chopped
- Extra-virgin olive oil
- Salt and black pepper to taste
- Paprika for garnish (optional)

Instructions

- Make sure to thoroughly clean the cucumbers. The ends should be trimmed and then cut into thick slices, with each slice measuring around half an inch to three quarters of an inch in thickness.
- Using a melon baller or a tiny spoon, carefully scoop out a small portion from the center of

each cucumber slice, creating a little well to hold the hummus.

- For the cucumber spaces, lightly sprinkle a mixture of salt and black pepper over the surface. The flavor of the cucumbers is enhanced by this particular process.

- A small amount of hummus should be poured into the well of each chamber of the cucumber. Ensure that the hummus is evenly distributed between the cups of cucumber.

- Every single cucumber hummus bite should be embellished with chopped fresh parsley, chopped cherry tomato halves, sliced Kalamata olives, crumbled feta cheese, and chopped fresh parsley. When it comes to the toppings, you are free to become creative.

- In order to add an additional layer of richness to the cucumber hummus bites, sprinkle a small amount of extra-virgin olive oil with a drizzler. There is a luxurious touch added by this step.

- At your discretion, you may choose to garnish the beverage with a sprinkling of paprika for color and a hint of smoke.

- It is recommended to arrange the Cucumber Hummuus Bite on a serving platter or board. Make sure that they are evenly placed in order to achieve a visually appealing presentation.

- Before serving, chill the bites in the refrigerator for fifteen to twenty minutes in order to provide a refreshment effect. This particular step serves to improve the crispness of the cucumbers.

- You can choose to indulge in a light and savory snack or provide these delectable bites to your guests on a regular basis. The crispness of the cucumber, the creaminess of the hummus, and the explosion of flavors from the toppings are all things that you should take pleasure in.

Guacamole with Jicama Slices

Ingredients

- 3 ripe avocados, peeled and pitted
- 1 small red onion, finely diced
- 2 medium tomatoes, diced
- 1/4 cup fresh cilantro, chopped
- 2 cloves garlic, minced
- 1 jalapeño, seeded and finely chopped (adjust according to spice preference)
- Juice of 1 lime
- Salt and black pepper to taste
- 1 large jicama, peeled and sliced into thin rounds or sticks

Instructions

- After placing the ripe avocado in a basin, use a fork to mash it, making sure to leave some chunks for texture.
- The mash avocado should be topped with finely chopped jalapeño, finely diced red

onion, and minced garlic. Stir in order to combine.

- Ensure that the diced tomatoes are evenly distributed throughout the guacamole by gently incorporating them into the mixture.

- It is recommended to squeeze the juice of one lime into the guacamole. The use of lime not only imparts a flavorful taste, but it also aids in preventing the swelling of the avodo.

- Ensure that the chopped cilantro is sprinkled over the guacamole layer. Combine thoroughly in order to incorporate the natural freshness of cilantro.

- Salt and black pepper should be added to the guacamole in accordance with your personal preferences in terms of flavor. Continue to mix in order to completely incorporate the spice.

- Take a taste of the guacamole and make any necessary adjustments to the lime, salt, or pepper. It is through this step that the ideal harmony of flavors is achieved.

- In order to prepare the jicama, peel it and then slice it into rounds or sticks. Because of its crisp texture, jicama offers a satisfying crunch and serves as a healthy alternative to tortilla chips.

- When arranging the jicama slices, make sure you do so on a serving platter or board. Place the bowl containing the guacamole in the middle of the serving arrangement after spooning it into the bowl.

- Ensure that the guacamole is finished with a garnish of additional cilantro or a sprinkling of paprika for an additional explosion of color and flavor.

- You may choose to invite your visitors to dip the jicama slices into the flavorful guacamole, or you may simply choose to enjoy this fresh and crunchy snack on your own personal time.

Roasted Red Pepper and Walnut Dip

Ingredients

- 2 large red bell peppers
- 2 tablespoons olive oil
- 2 cloves garlic, minced
- 4. 1 cup walnuts, toasted
- 1/4 cup breadcrumbs
- 2 tablespoons fresh lemon juice
- 2 tablespoons extra-virgin olive oil
- 1 teaspoon ground cumin
- 1/2 teaspoon smoked paprika
- Salt and black pepper to taste
- Fresh parsley or cilantro, chopped for garnish
- Pita bread or your favorite crackers

Instructions

- Make sure the oven's burner is preheated. It is recommended to place red bell peppers on a baking sheet and let them to roast, rotating them occasionally, until the skins become charred and blistered. This process takes approximately fifteen to twenty minutes.

- After the red peppers have been roasted, transfer them to a bowl and cover them with plastic wrap. Give them ten minutes to work together. After the peppers have been stalling, remove the seeded skin, peel off the charred skin, and chop the peppers.

- For approximately three to five minutes, or until the walnuts become a golden brown color, toast them in a dry skillet over a medium heat. It is important to avoid burning them. Take them away from the heat and let them to cool down.

- To prepare the dish, combine the toasted walnuts, breadcrumbs, lemon juice, extra-virgin olive oil, ground cumin, smoked paprika, salt, and black pepper in a food processor. Work the ingredients until it reaches the consistency of a coarse paste.

- You should incorporate the chopped roasted red peppers and minced garlic into the walnut mixture that is being processed in the food processor. Continue blending until the mixture is completely smooth and thoroughly combined.

- Taste the dip and make any necessary adjustments to the seasoning by adding additional salt, pepper, or lemon juice if necessary.

- In order to enhance the flavor, it is recommended to refrigerate the Roasted Red Pepper and Walnut Dip for a minimum of one hour prior to serving. As a result, the flavors are able to combine.

- If you want to add a splash of color and a hint of herbal aroma, garnish the dish with chopped fresh parsley or cilantro right before serving.

- Ensure that the dip is transferred to a bowl that is designated for serving. Ensure that you have a selection of crackers or pita bread available for dipping alongside.

- It is highly recommended that you invite your guests to indulge in the delicious and nutty goodness of this Roasted Red Pepper and

Walnut Dipped dish. As you savor each bite, take pleasure in the opulent flavors and velvety texture of the food.

Mixed Berry Parfait

Ingredients

- 2 cups mixed berries (strawberries, blueberries, raspberries, blackberries)
- 1/4 cup granulated sugar
- 1 tablespoon lemon juice
- 1 teaspoon cornstarch mixed with 1 tablespoon water (optional, for thickening)
- 2 cups Greek yogurt (or yogurt of your choice)
- 2 tablespoons honey or maple syrup
- 1 teaspoon vanilla extract
- 1 cup granola (store-bought or homemade)
- Extra mixed berries for garnish
- Fresh mint leaves for a touch of freshness

- The mixture of mixed berries, granulated sugar, and lemon juice should be combined in a saucepan. While the mixture is being cooked over medium heat, wait for the berries to release their juices and for the mixture to thicken slightly. It is possible to achieve a thicker consistency by adding the mixture of water and cornstarch, if desired. Take a break in order to cool off.

- Using a bowl, combine Greek yogurt with honey (or a simple syrup) and vanilla extract. Stir the mixture until it is thoroughly combined. You can adjust the sweetness to your preference.

- To begin, place a layer of the yogurt mixture that has been flavored with vanilla extract at the bottom of the serving glasses or bowls. In order to have a delicious crunch, you need follow this with a layer of granola.

- The granola should be topped with a layer of the mixed berry compote from the spoon. In order to create a visually appealing presentation, it is important to have an even distribution of berries. To do this, repeat the layering process by adding another layer of vanilla yogurt, then adding granola, and finally adding the berry compote. Maintain this process until you reach the highest point of the serving bowl or glass.

- Ensure that the parfait is topped with a substantial quantity of freshly mixed berries. The final presentation is enhanced with a blast of color and a sense of freshness thanks to this.

- PtsFresh mint leaves can be used to garnish the Mixed Berry Parfait, which will provide an additional touch of freshness to the dish.

- In order to allow the flavors to combine and the layers to settle, it is recommended to refrigerate the desserts for a minimum of one to two hours prior to serving.

- Dive into the layers of sweetness, creaminess, and crunchiness that each spoonful of this refreshing Mixed Berry Pastry brings to the table. The blend of flavors and textures is a delightful experience to behold.

Almond Flour Banana Bread

Ingredients

Dry Ingredients

- 2 cups almond flour
- 1/2 cup coconut flour
- 1 teaspoon baking soda
- 1/2 teaspoon baking powder
- 1/2 teaspoon salt

Wet Ingredients:

- 3 ripe bananas, mashed
- 3 large eggs
- 1/4 cup coconut oil, melted (or melted butter)
- 1/3 cup honey or maple syrup
- 1 teaspoon vanilla extract

Add-ins (Optional):

- 11. 1/2 cup chopped nuts (walnuts or pecans)
- 1/2 cup chocolate chips

Topping (Optional):

- Sliced bananas, additional nuts, or a sprinkle of cinnamon for garnish

Instructions

- The oven should be preheated to 350 degrees Fahrenheit (175 degrees Celsius). Prepare a standard loaf pan by greasing it and then lining it with parchment paper to facilitate easy removal.
- To make the batter, combine the following ingredients in a large mixing bowl: almond flour, coconut flour, baking soda, baking powder, and salt. Make sure that the dry ingredients are thoroughly mixed together.

- By utilizing a fork or a potato masher, the ripe bananas should be mashed in a separate bowl until they are smooth.

- You should incorporate the mashed bananas into the dry ingredients. Eggs, caramelized coconut oil (or butter), honey (or maple syrup), and vanilla extract should be included into the mixture. Mix the batter until it is completely smooth and well combined.

- If you desire to add texture and flavor to the batter, you can incorporate chopped nuts and chocolate chips into the base of the batter.

- Pour the batter into the loaf pan that has been prepared, making sure to distribute it evenly.

- To create a visually appealing toucch, you might choose to adorn the top with sliced bananas, extra nuts, or a sprinkling of cinnamon.

- The cake should be baked in the preheated oven for fifty to sixty minutes, or until a toothpick that is inserted into the center comes out clean. Be sure to keep a close eye on the bread and make adjustments as necessary, as baking times can vary.

- Allow the Almond Flour Banana Bread to cool in the pan for approximately fifteen minutes before transferring it to a wire rack to finish cooling completely. After it has cooled down, divide it into the desired amounts.

- It is recommended to serve the slices of Almond Flour Banana Bread either on their own or with a dollop of Greek yogurt or nut butter topping. Experiment with the most delicious and nuttiness!

Avocado Chocolate Mousse

Ingredients

Base

- 3 ripe avocados, peeled and pitted
- 1/2 cup unsweetened cocoa powder
- 1/2 cup pure maple syrup or honey
- 1/4 cup almond milk (or any milk of your choice)

- 1 teaspoon vanilla extract

Chocolate Addition:

- 1/2 cup dark chocolate, melted (70% cocoa or higher)

Optional Add-ins:

- A pinch of sea salt
- Espresso powder for a hint of coffee flavor
- 1-2 tablespoons nut butter (almond, peanut, or hazelnut)
- Fresh berries or mint leaves for garnish

Instructions

- Ensure that the avocadoes are in a state of ripeness. Take the fruit and toss it in a blender or food processor after you have scooped it out.
- Make sure to incorporate unsweetened cocoa powder into the blender or food processor.

Because of this, the chocolatey base of the fragrance is formed.

- Please incorporate pure maple syrup or honey into the mousse in order to naturally sweeten it. Set the sweetness level according to your liking.

- It is recommended to incorporate almond milk (or your preferred milk) in order to achieve a smooth consistency. This assists in achieving the desired texture of the moustache.

- The addition of vanilla essence provides a subtle hint of warmth and enhances the richness of flavor. Blend the ingredients until they are completely smooth.

- Put the dark chocolate in a heatproof bowl and place it over a double boiler. Alternatively, you can melt it in the microwave in short bursts. Stir the mixture until it becomes smooth, and then let it to cool down slowly.

- One should add the dark chocolate that has been melted into the avodo mixture. Repeat the process of blending until the mixture is completely incorporated, which will result in a luxurious and luscious fragrance.

- Enhance the flavor by adding a pinch of sea salt, espresso powder for a coffee twist, or incorporated nut butter for an additional layer of richness.

- When the texture of the mixture is too thick, you have the option of adding a little bit more almond milk and blending it until you achieve the desired consistency.

- It is recommended to transfer the Avvocado Chocolate Mouss to serving glasses or bowls and allow it to refrigerate for a minimum of two hours in order to allow it to cool down and improve the flavors.

- In order to bring forth an elegant presentation, it is recommended to garnish the mouth with fresh berries, mint leaves, or a dusting of cocoa powder prior to serving.

- I invite you to immerse yourself in the luxurious goodness of this guilt-free Avogado Chocolate Moussée. Embrace the velvety texture and the luscious chocolate flavor that each spoonful brings to the table.

Turkey and Cranberry Delight

Ingredients

- 1 pound ground turkey
- 1/2 cup breadcrumbs
- 1/4 cup grated Parmesan cheese
- 1/4 cup finely chopped onion
- 2 cloves garlic, minced
- 1 teaspoon dried sage
- 1 teaspoon dried thyme
- Salt and black pepper to taste
- 2 tablespoons olive oil (for cooking)

Cranberry Sauce:

- 1 cup fresh or frozen cranberries
- 1/2 cup orange juice
- 1/2 cup granulated sugar
- Zest of one orange
- 1 cinnamon stick (optional)

- 1/4 teaspoon ground ginger (optional)

- 4 slices of Brie or Camembert cheese

- 4 burger buns or slices of your favorite bread

- A handful of fresh arugula for garnish

Instructions

- The ground turkey, breadcrumbs, grated Parmesan cheese, chopped onion, minced garlic, dried sage, dried thyme, salt, and black pepper are all mixed together in a mixing bowl. Combine thoroughly until everything is incorporated.

- PtsIn order to create patties, divide the turkey mixture into four equal amounts and shape them into circles. Make sure that they are in a size that allows them to be cooked.

- To prepare the olive oil, heat it in a skillet over a medium heat. To ensure that the turkey patties are fully cooked and golden brown on the outside, grill them for a duration of five to six minutes per side. Ensure that they reach an internal temperature of 165 degrees Fahrenheit (74 degrees Celsius).

- Combine the following ingredients in a saucepan: cranberries, orange juice, granulated sugar, orange zest, cinnamon stick, and ground ginger. Initially, bring the mixture to a boil, and then reduce the heat and allow it to simmer for around ten to fifteen minutes, or until the canberries burst and the sauce becomes thick. Proceed to remove the cinnamon stick.

- In the final few minutes of cooking, it is recommended to apply a thin layer of butter or oil to each turkey patty in order to ensure that it melts smoothly.

- Ensure that the burger buns or slices of bread are toasted in a toaster or on a griddle until they are golden brown.

- On the bottom half of each bun, position a turkey patty that has melted butter or chocolate between the two halves. Spread a substantial quantity of cherry sauce all over the patty before serving.

- The addition of a handful of fresh arugula on top of the cherry sauce will provide a burst of freshness to the dish.

- In order to finish the sandwich, you should place the top half of the bun over the arugula.

- Take care of the cranberry and the turmeric. Please enjoy a deliciously warm meal, possibly accompanied by your preferred side dishes or a crisp salad.

- The combination of savoury turkey patties, the sweet-tartness of cherry sauce, and the creamy richness of either butter or camber in every bite is a delectable experience.

Grilled Salmon and Asparagus

Ingredients

Salmon Marinade

- 4 salmon fillets
- 2 tablespoons olive oil
- 2 tablespoons lemon juice
- 2 cloves garlic, minced

- 1 teaspoon dried dill

- Salt and black pepper to taste

- 1 bunch of fresh asparagus

- 1 tablespoon olive oil

- Salt and black pepper to taste

- Lemon Wedges (for Serving):

- Fresh lemon wedges for a citrusy finish

Instructions

- To prepare the marinade for the salad, combine olive oil, lemon juice, minced garlic, dried chili, salt, and black pepper in a bowl. Mix all of these ingredients together until fully combined.

- The salmon fillets should be placed in a low-sided dish and coated with the marinade until they are completely covered. Give the salmon a minimum of fifteen to thirty minutes to marinate in order for it to fully absorb the flavors.

- Raise the temperature of your grill to a medium-high level. In order to prevent the grates from sticking, it is important to ensure that they are thoroughly cleaned and lubricated.

- Ensure that the tough ends of the asparagus spears are trimmed. In a separate bowl, carefully combine the asparagus with olive oil, salt, and black pepper, ensuring that they are completely coated.

- Put the salmon fillets that have been marinated on the grill that has been preheated. For approximately four to five minutes on each side, or until the salmon is fully cooked and has a grill mark, grill the salmon. The duration of cooking time may differ depending on the thickness of the fillets.

- During the time that the salmon is being cooked, include the seasoned asparagus into the grill. Grill the asparagus for around five to seven minutes, turning it occasionally, until it becomes tender but maintains its crisp texture.

- If you want to check whether the salumin is finished, you can use a work to see if it breaks easily. The temperature inside should reach 145 degrees Fahrenheit (63 degrees Celsius).

- The grilled asparagus and the grilled salmon should be transferred to a serving platter. If there is any remaining marinade, drizzle it over the top.

- The dish should be garnished with fresh lemon wedges in order to get a zesty finish. When lemon juice is squeezed over almonds, the flavors of the almonds are enhanced.

- Ensure that the Grilled is served. Salmon and Asparagus are a combination that is both hot and savor, resembling the ideal combination of crisp asparagus and salmon.

Herb-Roasted Pork Tenderloin

Ingredients

- 2 pork tenderloins (about 1 to 1.5 pounds each)
- 3 tablespoons olive oil
- 3 cloves garlic, minced
- 1 tablespoon Dijon mustard
- 1 tablespoon balsamic vinegar
- 1 tablespoon soy sauce
- 1 tablespoon honey or maple syrup
- 1 teaspoon dried rosemary
- 1 teaspoon dried thyme
- 1 teaspoon dried sage
- Salt and black pepper to taste
- 1 teaspoon dried rosemary
- 1 teaspoon dried thyme
- 1 teaspoon dried sage
- 1 teaspoon garlic powder
- Salt and black pepper to taste
- Fresh parsley or rosemary for garnish

Instructions

- To make the marignade, combine olive oil, minced garlic, Dijon mustard, balsamic vinegar, soy sauce, honey (or maple syrup), dried rosemary, dried thyme, dried sage, salt, and black pepper in a bowl. Whisk all of these ingredients together until they are thoroughly combined.

- The pork tenderloins should be placed in a plastic bag that can be sealed or in a dish that can be sealed. Pour the marinade over the pork, making sure that it is distributed evenly throughout the surface. Marinate for a minimum of thirty minutes, or alternatively, refrigerate for two to four hours or overnight, in order to achieve the maximum flavor intensity.

- The oven should be preheated to 400 degrees Fahrenheit (200 degrees Celsius).

- For the purpose of preparing the herb rub, combine the following ingredients in a small bowl: dried rosemary, dried thyme, dried salt, garlic powder, salt, and black pepper.

- In order to alleviate excess marine, remove the pock ligaments from the marine and allow the excess marine to drain away. Serve the marinade for the purpose of basting.

- To get an even coating, rub the herb mixture over the surface of each planter, being sure to cover the entire surface.

- PtsTo enhance the flavor, heat a skillet over medium heat and sear the pork tendon slices for one to two minutes on each side until they are browned. Enjoy the enhanced flavor! Not only is this step optional, but it also contributes to the overall texture and flavor.

- It is recommended to position the pork tenderloins on a baking sheet or a roasting pan that has been lined with parchment paper. Roast in the oven that has been warmed for twenty to twenty-five minutes, or until the internal temperature reaches 145 degrees Fahrenheit (63 degrees Celsius), basting with the marine that has been served halfway through the cooking process.

- Please allow the roasted pork tenderloin to rest for a duration of five to ten minutes before to slicing it. In addition to ensuring a more soft and tender result, this helps to preserve the juices.

- To prepare the dish, cut the pork tenderloin into medallions and arrange them on a serving platter. If desired, garnish the dish with fresh parsley or rosemary.

- The Herb-Roasted Pork should be preserved. With tenderloin serving as the focal point of your meal, you may savor the harmonic blend of herbs and the scrumptiousness of perfectly roasted meat.

CONCLUSION

I have delved into the fundamentals of a low-sodium diet, discovered the secrets of a well-stocked kitchen, and delved into a variety of breakfasts, lunches, dinners, snacks, and special treats, all of which have been precisely crafted to maintain histamine levels in check while also appealing to your taste buds.

Through the use of this cookbook, you learned about histamine intolerance as well as the ways in which particular foods may influence our health. Having acquired the necessary information, I proceeded to explore the world of flavorings, low-sodium components, and the development of a wide variety of dishes that are appropriate for a variety of events.

Your health and happiness were taken into consideration when developing each and every recipe, from the stimulating smoothie bowls to the comforting lentil soups that can be made in a single pot.

In order to ensure that you are able to enjoy delectable meals regardless of the restrictions that you have placed on your diet, I investigated innovative approaches to traditional cuisine.

The construction of a low-height kitchen turned out to be an experience that was both amusing and educational. It allowed for the provision of useful advice on important ingredients and sensible selections. The journey proceeded to the breakfast table, lunchbox, dinner spread, and even special events, illustrating that a low-histamine way of life does not involve giving up taste or variety.

The adventure continued to the dinner spread. While you are enjoying these meals, it is important to keep in mind that adopting a low-hamine diet requires you to make choices that are not only flavorful but also beneficial to your health. The purpose of this cookbook is to encourage you to make your health a priority while also providing you with a wide range of delicious dishes.

The time you spend in your kitchen ought to be filled with joy, excitement, and the opportunity to try new things.

You are on the way to a diet that is low in histamines, and most importantly, you are looking for a source of nutrients that will make you happy, content, and inspired. With cheers, we celebrate the good health and tasty cuisine that we have found.